Carb Clarity

An Essential Guide to Making Wise Carb Choices for Healthy Living

By

Dr. Patricia Keller

Disclaimer

Copyright © 2023 by Dr Patricia Keller

This book is intended to provide helpful and informative material on the subject matter covered. It is not intended to serve as a substitute for professional medical advice or treatment. Any reliance you place on the information contained in this book is strictly at your own risk.

The author and publisher disclaim any liability for any injury or damage resulting from the use or misuse of the information presented in this book.

Table of Contents

Introduction

Carbohydrates are rich sources of macronutrients needed by the body to provide energy. However, with so much conflicting information about carbs in the media, it can be confusing to know how much to eat and which types are best for your health. Hence, the need for the book "Carb Clarity: An Essential Guide to Making Wise Carb Choices for Healthy Living."

In this book, we'll explore the science behind carbs and their different types, common myths about carbs, and the factors that influence your carb needs. You'll learn how to determine your carb tolerance, understand your metabolic type, and track your carb intake. We'll then dive into strategies for reducing carb intake, choosing the right carbs, and combining carbs with other macronutrients to support your health goals.

You'll also find practical tips for incorporating healthy carbs into your diet, such as meal and snack ideas, sample meal plans, and advice for eating out. Finally, we'll address common issues with carb intake, how to make adjustments to your carb intake, and how to deal with carb cravings.

With the information in this book, you'll be able to confidently customize your carb intake to support your health and wellness goals. So let's end the confusion and get started!

Chapter One

The Science of Carbs

Carbohydrates are one of the three macronutrients that provide energy to the body, along with fats and proteins. In this chapter, we'll explore the science behind carbs, including what they are, how they're digested, and how they affect your body.

What are Carbs?

Carbs, or carbohydrates, are molecules made up of carbon, hydrogen, and oxygen atoms. They come in different forms, including sugars, starches, and fiber. Many food sources contain carbs, some of which are dairy products, fruits, grains, and vegetables.

How are Carbs Digested?

When you eat carbs, your body breaks them down into glucose, a simple sugar that is used by cells for energy. Glucose is transported from the intestines into the bloodstream, where it is carried to cells throughout the body.

Insulin, a hormone produced by the pancreas, helps transport glucose into cells. If you eat more carbs than your body needs for energy, the excess glucose is stored in the liver and muscles as glycogen. When your body needs energy, it can break down glycogen into glucose and use it for fuel.

How do Carbs Affect Your Body?

Carbs are the body's primary source of energy, and they play a critical role in brain function, muscle function, and maintaining a healthy weight. However, carbs function in different ways.

Simple carbs, like those found in sugary drinks and processed foods, are quickly digested and can cause a rapid spike in blood sugar levels. This can lead to a crash in energy and increased hunger and cravings.

Complex carbs, which do not digest easily contain great sources of energy examples are whole grains, vegetables, and fruits. They also contain fiber, which can help regulate blood sugar levels and promote feelings of fullness.

Common Myths About Carbs

Carbs are often the subject of controversy and confusion in the nutrition world. In this chapter, we'll explore some of the common myths about carbs and provide evidence-based information to help you make informed decisions about your carb intake.

Myth: All carbs are bad for you.
Fact: Not all carbs are created equal. While simple carbs like refined sugars and white flour can have negative effects on the body, complex carbs like whole grains, fruits, and vegetables provide important nutrients and are essential for a healthy diet.

Myth: Carbs make you gain weight.

Fact: Consuming excess calories from any source, including carbs, can lead to weight gain. However, carbs can also provide a source of energy for physical activity and can help you feel full and satisfied, which can support weight loss goals.

Myth: Weight Loss can only be achieved through a low-carb diet.

Fact: Low-carb diets can lead to weight loss, but they are not the only or necessarily the best approach. A balanced diet that includes a variety of foods, including complex carbs, can support long-term weight loss and overall health.

Myth: Carbs cause diabetes.

Fact: While consuming excess calories from any source can lead to weight gain, there is no evidence to support the idea that carbs, in and of themselves, cause diabetes. Complex carbs can help regulate blood sugar levels and reduce the risk of type 2 diabetes.

Myth: You need to cut out carbs to be healthy.

Fact: Carbs are an essential part of a healthy diet and provide important nutrients like fiber, vitamins, and minerals. Cutting out carbs entirely can lead to nutrient deficiencies and have negative effects on health.

By dispelling these common myths, you can make informed decisions about your carb intake and achieve optimal health. In the next chapter, we'll explore how to assess your carb needs and determine the right balance of carbs for your body.

Chapter Two

Assessing Your Carb Needs

When it comes to customizing your carb intake, it's important to assess your individual needs. In this chapter, we'll cover several factors that can influence your carb needs, including:

- How to Determine Your Carb Tolerance: We'll explain what carb tolerance is and how to figure out your carb tolerance level, as well as what to do if you're not sure.
- Factors That Influence Your Carb Needs: We'll discuss how factors such as age, gender, activity level, and health conditions can impact your carb needs.
- Understanding Your Metabolic Type: We'll explore the concept of metabolic typing and how it can help you determine the best carb intake for your body.
- Tracking Your Carb Intake: We'll explain how tracking your carb intake can help you assess your carb needs and make adjustments as necessary.

By the end of this chapter, you'll have a better understanding of your individual carb needs and how to customize your carb intake for optimal health.

How to Determine Your Carb Tolerance

To determine your carb tolerance, you'll need to pay attention to how your body reacts to different amounts of carbohydrates. Here are some steps you can take to figure out your carb tolerance level:

Start with a moderate carb intake: Begin by consuming a moderate amount of carbohydrates, such as 100-150 grams per day. This will be your starting point.

Be conscious of your energy levels: How you feel throughout the day should be observed. Do you have sustained energy or do you experience energy crashes?

Observe your hunger levels: Take note of how hungry you feel throughout the day. Are you able to go several hours between meals or do you find yourself snacking frequently?

Monitor your weight: Keep track of your weight to see if you're gaining or losing weight at this carb intake level.

Adjust as necessary: If you feel good and are maintaining a healthy weight, your current carb intake is likely a good fit for your body. However, if you're experiencing energy crashes or are not seeing the results you want, you may need to adjust your carb intake up or down.

It's important to remember that carb tolerance can vary greatly from person to person, and what works for one person may not work for another. Be patient and persistent in finding the carb intake that works best for you.

Factors That Influence Your Carb Needs

Several factors can influence your carb needs, including:

Age: As you age, your body becomes less efficient at processing carbohydrates, so you may need to reduce your carb intake as you get older.

Gender: Men tend to have higher carb needs than women, due to their larger body size and muscle mass.

Activity level: If you're very active and engage in regular exercise or physical labor, you may need more carbohydrates to fuel your body.

Health conditions: Certain health conditions, such as diabetes or insulin resistance, may require you to limit your carb intake.

Genetics: Some people may be genetically predisposed to metabolize carbohydrates differently than others.

Stress levels: High levels of stress can affect your body's ability to process carbohydrates, so if you're under a lot of stress, you may need to reduce your carb intake.

Sleep patterns: Poor sleep can lead to insulin resistance and carb intolerance, so getting enough restful sleep is important for managing your carb needs.

The above-listed factors will give you an in-depth understanding of your personal carbs needs and make necessary adjustments to your carb consumption. It's also a good idea to consult with a healthcare professional if you have any underlying health conditions or concerns about your carb intake.

Understanding Your Metabolic Type

Understanding your metabolic type can help you determine how your body processes different types of macronutrients, including carbohydrates. Here are some of the different metabolic types:

Carbohydrate Efficient: People who are carbohydrate efficient tend to do well on diets that are higher in carbohydrates and lower in fat. They can process carbohydrates efficiently and may struggle with weight gain or other health issues when consuming a high-fat diet.

Protein Efficient: Protein-efficient individuals tend to do better on diets that are higher in protein and lower in carbohydrates. They may have trouble losing weight or may experience energy crashes when consuming a diet high in carbohydrates.

Mixed: Some people have a mixed metabolic type, meaning that they have characteristics of both carbohydrate-efficient and protein-efficient individuals. They may do well on a balanced diet that includes moderate amounts of all three macronutrients (carbohydrates, protein, and fat).

Balanced: Finally, some people have a balanced metabolic type, meaning that they can tolerate a wide range of macronutrient ratios and do not have any specific dietary requirements.

To determine your metabolic type, you can work with a healthcare professional or a qualified nutritionist who can assess your individual needs and provide personalized recommendations for your diet. By understanding your metabolic type, you can make more informed decisions about your carbohydrate intake and other dietary choices.

Tracking Your Carb Intake

Tracking your carb intake can be a useful tool for managing your diet and achieving your health goals. Here are some tips for tracking your carb intake:

Use a food diary: Keep a record of everything you eat and drink, including the portion sizes and carb content. Some many apps and websites can help you track your intake, or you can use a pen and paper.

Read food labels: Be aware of the carb content in the foods you consume, and read nutrition labels carefully to understand the carb content per serving.

Measure your portions: Use measuring cups and spoons to measure out your food portions and ensure that you're not accidentally over-consuming carbs.

Know your carb goals: Determine your daily carb goal based on your individual needs and goals, and adjust your intake accordingly.

Be consistent: Try to track your carb intake consistently every day to get an accurate picture of your intake and progress over time.

Be mindful: Pay attention to how your body responds to different levels of carb intake, and adjust your intake as needed based on your energy levels, mood, and other factors.

By tracking your carb intake, you can identify patterns in your diet and make informed decisions about your food choices to optimize your health and well-being.

Chapter Three

Customizing Your Carb Intake

This chapter focuses on customizing your carb intake based on your individual needs and goals. Here are some strategies for customizing your carb intake:

Determine your carb tolerance: Based on your metabolic type, lifestyle, and other factors, determine how many carbohydrates you can consume per day without negatively impacting your health or weight loss goals.

Choose the right carbs: Not all carbs are created equal. Choose complex, whole-food sources of carbs like fruits, vegetables, and whole grains, and avoid processed and refined carbs like sugary drinks, baked goods, and white bread.

Time your carb intake strategically: Consider timing your carb intake around your workouts or other physical activities to provide energy and support recovery.

Incorporate healthy fats and proteins: Pairing healthy fats and proteins with your carbs can help slow down digestion and promote satiety, helping you feel full and satisfied for longer.

Experiment with carb cycling: Some people find that alternating between higher-carb and lower-carb days can help support their energy levels, weight loss goals, and overall health.

By customizing your carb intake based on your individual needs and goals, you can optimize your diet and achieve optimal health and well-being. It's important to work with a healthcare professional or qualified nutritionist to determine the best approach for your individual needs.

Strategies for Reducing Carb Intake

Reducing carb intake can be a helpful strategy for managing blood sugar levels, promoting weight loss, and improving overall health. Here are some strategies for reducing carb intake:

Swap out high-carb foods for low-carb alternatives: Instead of bread, pasta, and rice, try substituting with low-carb options like zucchini noodles, cauliflower rice, or lettuce wraps.

Focus on protein and healthy fats: Incorporating more protein and healthy fats in your meals can help keep you feeling full and satisfied, while also supporting muscle growth and repair.

Increase vegetable intake: Vegetables are a great source of fiber, vitamins, and minerals, and can help fill you up without adding a lot of extra carbs.

Reduce or eliminate sugary drinks: Soda, juice, and other sugary drinks can add a lot of extra carbs and calories to your diet. Try replacing them with water, herbal tea, or other low-carb options.

Plan: Planning your meals and snacks ahead of time can help you make healthier choices and avoid reaching for high-carb options out of convenience.

Remember that everyone's carb needs and tolerances are different, so it's important to work with a healthcare professional or qualified nutritionist to determine the best approach for your individual needs.

Choosing the Right Carbs

Choosing the right types of carbs can make a big difference in your overall health and well-being. When choosing the right carbs, the following should be looked into:

Look for whole-food sources: Whole-food sources of carbs, such as fruits, vegetables, and whole grains, are generally more nutrient-dense and provide a variety of vitamins, minerals, and fiber.

Avoid refined and processed carbs: Refined and processed carbs, such as white bread, pasta, and sugary snacks, are often stripped of important nutrients and can spike blood sugar levels, leading to energy crashes and cravings.

Focus on fiber: High-fiber carbs, such as leafy greens, berries, and whole grains, can help promote feelings of fullness, improve digestion, and support healthy blood sugar levels.

Consider glycemic load: The glycemic load is a measure of how quickly a food raises blood sugar levels. Choosing lower glycemic load carbs, such as sweet potatoes, quinoa, and lentils, can help support stable energy levels and prevent blood sugar spikes.

Pay attention to portion sizes: Even healthy carbs can add up quickly, so it's important to pay attention to portion sizes and balance your carb intake with protein, healthy fats, and non-starchy vegetables.

By choosing the right types of carbs and balancing your carb intake with other nutrients, you can support your overall health and well-being. Remember to work with a healthcare professional or qualified nutritionist to determine the best approach for your individual needs.

Chapter Four

Combining Carbs with Other Macronutrients

When it comes to optimal health and nutrition, it's not just about the types of carbs you choose, but also how you combine them with other macronutrients. Here are some tips for combining carbs with other nutrients:

Pair carbs with protein: Combining carbs with protein can help slow down the absorption of sugar into the bloodstream, preventing blood sugar spikes and promoting satiety. Examples of carb-protein combinations include apple slices with almond butter or a quinoa and vegetable stir-fry with chicken.

Add healthy fats: Adding healthy fats to your carb-containing meals can also help slow down digestion and keep you feeling fuller for longer. Examples of carb-fat combinations include avocado toast with a poached egg or a spinach salad with olive oil and almonds.

Balance your plate: When planning your meals, aim to fill half your plate with non-starchy vegetables, one quarter with protein, and one-quarter with healthy carbs. This can help ensure you're getting a variety of nutrients and supporting healthy blood sugar levels.

Timing is key: It's also important to consider the timing of your carb intake. Consuming carbs before or after exercise can help support energy levels and muscle recovery while consuming carbs before bed can promote restful sleep and help regulate hunger hormones.

By combining carbs with protein, healthy fats, and non-starchy vegetables, you can support healthy digestion, blood sugar levels, and overall health and well-being. Remember to work with a healthcare professional or qualified nutritionist to determine the best approach for your individual needs.

Pairing Carbs with Protein

Pairing carbs with protein is a great way to balance your meals and support optimal health. Here's why:

Slows down digestion: When you eat carbs alone, they are quickly broken down into glucose and absorbed into your bloodstream, leading to a rapid rise in blood sugar levels. However, when you pair carbs with protein, the protein helps slow down the absorption of glucose into your bloodstream, preventing blood sugar spikes and promoting stable energy levels.

Promotes satiety: Protein is also more filling than carbs, so by pairing the two, you are likely to feel fuller for longer and less likely to overeat.

Provides essential nutrients: Pairing carbs with protein can also help ensure you are getting a balance of essential nutrients. For example, pairing brown rice with grilled chicken provides both carbohydrates for energy and protein for muscle repair and growth.

Examples of carb-protein combinations include:

- Greek yogurt with berries

- Apple slices with almond butter

- Hummus with carrots and whole-grain pita

- Grilled chicken with roasted sweet potatoes

- Quinoa and vegetable stir-fry with tofu

Remember, the key is to choose healthy sources of carbs and protein, such as whole grains, fruits, vegetables, lean meats, legumes, and nuts, and to balance your meals to support optimal health and well-being.

Adding Healthy Fats to Your Carb-Containing Meals

Adding healthy fats to your carb-containing meals is another way to support optimal health and promote satiety. Here's why:

Slows down digestion: Just like protein, fat can also help slow down the digestion and absorption of carbs, preventing blood sugar spikes and promoting stable energy levels.

Increases satiety: Fats take longer to digest than carbs or protein, which means they can help keep you feeling fuller for longer and less likely to overeat.

Provides essential nutrients: Healthy fats, such as those found in avocados, nuts, seeds, and olive oil, provide essential nutrients like omega-3 and omega-6 fatty acids, vitamin E, and antioxidants.

Examples of carb-fat combinations include:

- Oatmeal with almond butter and sliced banana

- Barbequed salmon with simmered sweet potatoes and asparagus

- Whole-grain toast with avocado and scrambled eggs

- Quinoa salad with mixed veggies and a drizzle of olive oil

- Greek yogurt with blended berries and cleaved nuts

Remember, the key is to choose healthy sources of fats, such as those found in nuts, seeds, avocados, olive oil, and fatty fish, and to balance your meals with a mix of carbs, protein, and fats to support optimal health and well-being.

Being Mindful of Portion Sizes

Being mindful of portion sizes is an important aspect of customizing your carb intake for optimal health. The following tips to help you keep track of your portions:

Use measuring cups and spoons: Measuring cups and spoons can help you accurately portion out your carbs and prevent overeating.

Visualize portion sizes: Use everyday objects as visual cues to help you estimate portion sizes. For example, a serving of fruit is roughly the size of a tennis ball, while a serving of rice or pasta is about the size of a closed fist.

Don't eat straight from the bag or container: Eating straight from the bag or container can make it easy to lose track of how much you've eaten. Instead, portion out your carbs onto a plate or bowl before eating.

Listen to your body: Pay attention to how you feel during and after meals. If you feel overly full or uncomfortable, you may have eaten too much.

Remember, everyone's portion needs are different, so it's important to listen to your body and adjust your portions accordingly. By being mindful of portion sizes, you can enjoy your favorite carbs while still supporting your health and well-being.

Considering the Timing of Your Carb Intake

Considering the timing of your carb intake can also be important for optimizing your health. Here are some tips to help you time your carb intake effectively:

Eat most of your carbs earlier in the day: Consuming the bulk of your carbs earlier in the day can help provide you with energy throughout the day and prevent overeating later in the day.

Time your carbs around your workouts: Consuming carbs before and after exercise can help fuel your workouts and support recovery.

Limit carbs at night: Consuming large amounts of carbs at night can disrupt sleep and contribute to weight gain. Instead, focus on eating a protein-rich dinner with a moderate amount of carbs.

Consider your individual needs: Everyone's carb timing needs may differ depending on their activity level, metabolism, and other factors. Test a series of timing strategies to find the most suitable one for you.

Remember, while the timing of your carb intake can be important, it's also important to focus on overall carb quality and quantity. By incorporating a variety of healthy, whole-food carbs into your diet and balancing them with protein and healthy fats, you can support optimal health and well-being.

Chapter Five

Incorporating Healthy Carbs into Your Diet

In this chapter, we will explore the various healthy carb sources that you can incorporate into your diet for optimal health. Here are some examples:

Whole grains: Whole grains are a great source of healthy carbs, fiber, and nutrients. Examples include brown rice, quinoa, oatmeal, and whole wheat bread.

Fruits: Fruits are not only delicious but also packed with vitamins, minerals, and antioxidants. Some examples of healthy fruits include berries, apples, oranges, and bananas.

Vegetables: Vegetables are also an excellent source of healthy carbs, fiber, and nutrients. Leafy greens, carrots, peppers, and sweet potatoes are just a few examples of healthy vegetables you can incorporate into your diet.

Legumes: Legumes, such as lentils, beans, and chickpeas, are another great source of healthy carbs, fiber, and plant-based protein.

Nuts and seeds: Nuts and seeds are not only a great source of healthy fats but also provide a good amount of healthy carbs. Almonds, chia seeds, and pumpkin seeds are good sources of healthy carbs.

Incorporating a variety of these healthy carb sources into your diet can provide you with the energy and nutrients your body needs to thrive. It's also important to focus on balance and portion control to ensure that you're getting the right amount of carbs for your individual needs.

Tips for Choosing Healthy Carbs

Sure! Here are some factors for selecting healthy carbs:

Look for complex carbs: Complex carbs are digested slowly, which means they provide a steady source of energy and keep you feeling full for longer. Sources of complex carbs include fruits, vegetables and whole grains.

Avoid refined carbs: Refined carbs, such as white bread, pasta, and sugar, are digested quickly and can cause spikes in blood sugar levels. They also lack the nutrients found in whole, unrefined carbs.

Read food labels: When selecting packaged foods, check the label for added sugars and refined carbs. Look for products that are high in fiber and have a low glycemic index.

Focus on variety: Incorporating a variety of healthy carbs into your diet ensures that you are getting a range of essential nutrients.

Practice portion control: While healthy carbs can provide important nutrients, it's important to practice portion control to avoid overconsumption. Aim for a balance of healthy carbs, protein, and healthy fats at each meal.

By following these tips, you can make informed choices when it comes to incorporating healthy carbs into your diet.

Healthy Carb-Containing Meal Ideas

Sure, here are some healthy carb-containing meal ideas:

Quinoa salad with mixed vegetables, avocado, and grilled chicken: Quinoa is a great source of complex carbs and protein, while vegetables and avocado provide additional fiber and healthy fats.

Whole wheat pasta with marinara sauce, sautéed spinach, and turkey meatballs: Whole wheat pasta provides complex carbs and fiber, while the turkey meatballs offer a source of lean protein.

Brown rice bowl with roasted sweet potato, black beans, and salsa: Brown rice is a nutritious complex carb, while sweet potatoes and black beans provide additional fiber, vitamins, and minerals. Salsa adds flavor and is a low-calorie source of vegetables.

Oatmeal with mixed berries, nuts, and cinnamon: Oatmeal is a filling source of complex carbs and fiber, while berries and nuts provide additional antioxidants and healthy fats. Cinnamon adds flavor and can help regulate blood sugar levels.

Chickpea and vegetable stir-fry with brown rice: Chickpeas are a great source of plant-based protein and complex carbs, while vegetables offer fiber and vitamins. Brown rice provides additional complex carbs and fiber.

These meal ideas are just a starting point – there are endless ways to incorporate healthy carbs into your diet!

Sample Meal Plans:

Here are three sample meal plans that incorporate healthy carbs:

Breakfast: Greek yogurt with blended berries and granola
Lunch: Whole grain wrap with turkey, avocado, spinach, and hummus
Dinner: Barbecued salmon with simmered sweet potato and asparagus

Breakfast: Oatmeal with sliced banana and almond butter
Lunch: Grilled chicken with quinoa and roasted vegetables
Dinner: Vegetable stir-fry with brown rice and tofu

Breakfast: Whole grain toast with avocado and poached egg
Lunch: Lentil soup with whole grain crackers and mixed greens salad
Dinner: Baked sweet potato with black bean chili and a side salad

Snack Ideas

Sure, here are some healthy snack ideas that include carbs:

Apple slices with almond butter: Apples provide fiber and vitamins, while almond butter offers a source of healthy fats and protein.

Greek yogurt with blended berries and granola: Greek yogurt provides protein and carbs, while berries offer antioxidants and fiber. Granola provides additional carbs and texture.

Hummus and vegetable sticks: Hummus is made from chickpeas, which provide protein and complex carbs. Vegetables offer fiber and vitamins.

Rice cakes with avocado and cherry tomatoes: Rice cakes are a low-calorie source of complex carbs, while avocado offers healthy fats and fiber. Cherry tomatoes add flavor and additional nutrients.

Trail mix with dried fruit and nuts: Dried fruit provides carbs and fiber, while nuts offer a source of healthy fats and protein. Just make sure to choose a trail mix that isn't loaded with added sugars.

These snack ideas are just a few examples – there are plenty of other healthy carb-containing snacks out there!

Tips for Eating Out

Sure, here are some tips for eating out while still being mindful of your carb intake:

Check the menu ahead of time: Many restaurants offer their menus online, so take a look before you go. This can help you plan and choose a dish that fits within your carb goals.

Ask for substitutions: Many restaurants are happy to accommodate requests for substitutions or modifications. For example, you could ask for a side salad instead of fries or a bun-less burger.

Choose dishes with lots of vegetables: Vegetables are typically low in carbs and high in nutrients, so look for dishes that include plenty of veggies. For example, a stir-fry with lots of veggies and a protein source can be a great option.

Be mindful of portion sizes: Restaurant portions are often much larger than what you would serve yourself at home. Consider asking for a to-go container and packing up half of your meal to save for later.

Don't be afraid to ask questions: If you're not sure about a dish's ingredients or how it's prepared, don't be afraid to ask your server. They provide more tips and information to enable you to make wise decisions.

By following these tips, you can enjoy eating out without sacrificing your carb goals.

Chapter Six

Troubleshooting Your Carb Intake

Carb intake can be a tricky thing to navigate, and even with careful planning and tracking, sometimes things can go awry. Here are some common issues that people encounter with their carb intake, and some strategies for addressing them.

Common issues with Carb Intake

In this chapter, we'll discuss some common issues people may encounter when adjusting their carb intake and provide some troubleshooting tips:

Not Seeing Results: Sometimes, people may not see the desired results despite making changes to their carb intake. We'll explore potential reasons for this and provide solutions.

Digestive Issues: Some people may experience digestive issues when adjusting their carb intake. We'll discuss why this happens and ways to alleviate these issues.

Cravings and Hunger: Changing your carb intake can affect your appetite and cravings. We'll provide strategies to help manage hunger and cravings.

Energy and Performance: Carbs are an important source of energy for the body, and adjusting your intake can impact your energy levels and athletic performance. We'll discuss how to optimize your carb intake for optimal energy and performance.

Adapting to a Low-Carb Diet: For those transitioning to a low-carb diet, there may be an adjustment period. We'll provide tips for making this transition as smooth as possible.

How to Make Adjustments to Your Carb Intake

In this section, we'll explore how to make adjustments to your carb intake:

Gradual Changes: Making gradual changes to your carb intake is often the best approach. This allows your body to adjust slowly and can help prevent some of the issues that may arise from sudden changes.

Be Mindful of Your Progress: Be conscious of how you feel and any changes you observe. This can help you make informed decisions about adjusting your carb intake.

Experiment with Different Amounts and Types of Carbs: Everyone's carb needs and tolerances are different. Experimenting with different amounts and types of carbs can help you find what works best for your body.

Consider Your Activity Level: Your activity level can play a significant role in how many carbs you need. If you're extremely active, you may need more carbs than someone inactive.

Consult with a Healthcare Professional: If you have a medical condition or are on medication, it's important to consult with a healthcare professional before making any changes to your carb intake.

By following these guidelines, you can make informed decisions about your carb intake and optimize your health and well-being.

Dealing with Carb Cravings

Carb cravings can be difficult to deal with, but there are strategies you can use to help manage them:

Eat Regularly: Eating regular meals can help keep your blood sugar stable and prevent cravings. Try to eat every 3-4 hours to keep your body fueled and satisfied.

Focus on Protein and Healthy Fats: Protein and healthy fats can help keep you feeling full and satisfied, which can reduce cravings for carbs. Try to include these in every meal and snack.

Choose Complex Carbs: Complex carbs, such as whole grains, fruits, and vegetables, can provide sustained energy and help prevent cravings. Avoid simple carbs, such as sugary snacks and processed foods, which can cause blood sugar spikes and crashes.

Practice Careful Eating: Focus on your craving and fullness signs, and eat gradually and carefully. This can assist you with checking out your body's requirements and avoiding overheating.

Find Alternative Ways to Cope with Stress: Many people turn to carbs when they're stressed or anxious. Finding alternative ways to cope with stress, such as exercise or meditation, can help reduce cravings.

By incorporating these strategies into your daily routine, you can manage carb cravings and feel more in control of your diet and overall health.

Conclusion

In conclusion, carbohydrates play a significant role in our overall health and well-being, but it can be challenging to determine the right amount and type of carbs to consume. By understanding your carb needs, tracking your intake, and customizing your carb intake to your metabolic type, you can optimize your health and reduce the risk of chronic diseases. Incorporating healthy carbs into your diet, combining them with other macronutrients, and being mindful of portion sizes and timing can further enhance the benefits of carb consumption. And if you encounter issues with your carb intake, such as cravings or digestive problems, there are strategies and adjustments you can make to overcome them. With the knowledge and tools provided in this book, you can clarify your carb needs and achieve optimal health through a personalized approach to carb intake.

Summary of Key Takeaways

Here are some key takeaways from the book "Carb Clarity: An Essential Guide to Making Wise Carb Choices for Healthy Living."

- Carbohydrates are important macronutrients that provide energy and nutrients to the body.

- Not all carbs are created equal, and it's important to choose healthy carb sources such as fruits, vegetables, whole grains, and legumes.

- Assessing your carb needs based on your metabolic type, activity level, and other factors can help you determine the right amount of carbs to consume.

- Tracking your carb intake and being mindful of portion sizes and timing can help you achieve optimal health and reduce the risk of chronic diseases.

- Combining carbs with other macronutrients such as protein and healthy fats can enhance their benefits and promote satiety.

- Troubleshooting issues with your carb intake, such as cravings or digestive problems, requires adjustments and strategies that are personalized to your needs.

By following the strategies and recommendations provided in this book, you can clarify your carb needs and achieve optimal health through a customized approach to carb intake.

Tips for long-term success

In this book, we've covered a lot of ground when it comes to carbs and how they impact our health. Here are some tips for long-term success in customizing your carb intake:

Set realistic goals: Make sure your goals are achievable and sustainable in the long term. Gradual changes have a long-term effect, unlike drastic changes which do not last.

Experiment with different approaches: Everyone's body is different, so what works for one person may not work for another. Explore different approaches to finding what turns out best for you.

Focus on whole, nutrient-dense foods: Choose carbs that are whole and minimally processed, like fruits, vegetables, whole grains, and legumes. These foods provide more nutrients and fiber than highly processed carbs.

Don't forget about other macronutrients: While carbs are important, it's also important to make sure you're getting enough protein and healthy fats.

Be mindful of portion sizes: Even healthy carbs can contribute to weight gain if consumed in excess. Focus on portion measurements and adjust when necessary.

Keep track of your progress: Regularly check in with yourself and track your progress. Appreciate your progress and make the necessary adjustments.

By following these tips and keep educating yourself about carbs and their impact on health, you can achieve long-term success in customizing your carb intake for optimal health.

www.ingramcontent.com/pod-product-compliance
Lightning Source LLC
Chambersburg PA
CBHW061545250726
48657CB00006B/2301